The Surrogacy Solution:

A Complete Handbook on Becoming a Parent via Third-Party Procreation

By

Kimberly J. Bogle

Table of Content

Introduction

The Surrogacy Alternative

The want for a family is one of the most profoundly ingrained desires in the complex tapestry of the human experience. The desire to become a parent has long been a fundamental aspect of human existence, an innate urge that cuts beyond boundaries, countries, and even time. But the conventional routes to motherhood have taken on new shapes in today's world of changing family relations, bringing with them opportunities as well as obstacles that call for creative solutions.

In the middle of this changing environment, surrogacy has become a ray of light for single people and couples trying to figure out how to have a family. Surrogacy goes well beyond a simple medical treatment; it is a solution that provides a door to motherhood where other approaches might not work. It is a profound convergence of research, morality, and human connection. In the pages that follow, we take you on a trip into the core of this game-changing answer, delving into all of its facets. This book serves as a thorough manual a kind of road map for negotiating the surrogacy market with compassion, assurance, and clarity.

The fundamental message of "The Surrogacy Solution: A Complete Handbook on Becoming a Parent via Third Party Procreation", is that love has no boundaries and that the human spirit is resilient. It's a celebration of the varied fabric of contemporary families that surrogacy has contributed to weave, encompassing both same-sex couples hoping for their own child and individuals dealing with seemingly insurmountable infertility issues.

This book shows the way forward for the people who embrace the dream of becoming parents via the prism of personal stories, professional insights, and helpful advice. That journey is full of obstacles but also hope, possibilities, and the promise of an unending love. At its core, surrogacy is a singular combination of compassion, science, and the steadfast human urge to create and nurture life. Here are a few main explanations for why surrogacy is frequently accepted as a remedy:

Overcoming Infertility: Being infertile can be a significant obstacle to starting a family for many aspiring parents. Conventional techniques of conception may not work because of health issues, genetics, or other difficulties. Despite biological barriers, surrogacy provides a route forward so that people and couples can fulfill their goals of becoming parents.

Increasing Options for LGBTQ+ Families: For LGBTQ+ people and couples looking to start a family, surrogacy has been a game-changer. Particularly same-sex couples may use surrogacy to become biological parents, giving them the opportunity to enjoy the benefits of genetic relatedness and biological heritage in a manner that was previously unfeasible.

Genetic link: A special chance for intended parents and their kid to have a genetic link is offered by surrogacy. A surrogate provides the opportunity to preserve biological links while still going through the experience of pregnancy and labor in situations where one or both intended parents are unable to carry a pregnancy to term.

Medical Necessity: Surrogacy may be a necessary medical remedy in cases where pregnancy offers serious health hazards to the intended parent or parents, as well as the unborn child. To safely take the pregnancy to term, conditions including abnormalities in the uterus, a history of miscarriages, or grave worries about the health of the mother may need the use of a surrogate.

Choice and Autonomy: Surrogacy gives people the freedom to decide for themselves what kind of family to start. In contrast to adoption, which could require navigating convoluted legal and administrative procedures, surrogacy enables intended parents to actively participate in the whole pregnancy and delivery process.

Emotional Support and Connection: Deep emotional bonds are frequently forged between intended parents and their surrogate during the surrogacy process. A strong friendship can form via honest communication, respect for one another, and shared experiences, which will enhance the journey for all people involved.

Legal Protection: In countries with strict regulations governing surrogacy, legal frameworks offer protection and clarity to all parties. Everyone benefits from a smooth and safe process when there are clear agreements, rights that are defined, and legal recognition of parentage.

Global Accessibility: Thanks to technological developments and increased globalization, surrogacy is now more widely available to individuals and couples worldwide. Surrogacy reaffirms the great fact that love knows no bounds and offers those who dare to dream of motherhood opportunity, choice, and the potential of family fulfillment.

Come along as we explore the core of the surrogacy experience, where families are formed, miracles occur, and the whole complexity and beauty of what it means to produce life is revealed. Welcome to " **The Surrogacy Solution: A Complete Handbook on Becoming a Parent via Third-Party Procreation,**" where each page demonstrates how love has the ability to transform life itself.

Chapter 1

Understanding Surrogacy

The term "surrogacy," which was long relegated to the periphery of social discourse, has now become a mainstay in discussions about contemporary family formation. However, the idea is still cloaked in mystery, false beliefs, and unsolved concerns for a large number of people. This first chapter takes us on a voyage of exploration into the core of surrogacy, dissecting its characteristics, revealing its complexities, and illuminating the true nature of the practice.

As a means of expanding families, surrogacy is developing quickly. In 2019, 5.4% of all operations involving in vitro fertilization (IVF) involved surrogates. Why? With a 75% success rate, surrogacy is the most effective treatment for infertility. For a birth, that percentage can rise to 95% if the gestational carrier becomes pregnant.

What is Surrogacy?

A woman can become a surrogate by carrying a baby for another person or couple. Surrogacy is a contemporary and expanding method of starting a family. To transfer their embryo into the surrogate's uterus, the intended parents use in vitro fertilization, or IVF. More than 17,000 births in the US were surrogate mothers' babies in 2019, and the market is expected to increase at a rate of 15% annually. Furthermore, the proportion of all IVF transfers that used a gestational carrier increased by more than five times in the last ten years, from slightly over 1% to 5.4%.

A woman who becomes a surrogate, also known as a gestational carrier, bears a child on behalf of an individual or couple with whom she has no genetic link. The intended parent is the individual who is attempting to conceive using the surrogate. The intended parent(s) reimburses the surrogate for her time and expenses. The intended mother's egg, or donor egg, and the intended father's sperm, or donor sperm, combine to form the embryo. The intended parents take full responsibility for the kid and are identified as the legal parents on the birth certificate after the child is born. Misconceptions regarding gestational carriers, often known as surrogates, are common.

A gestational surrogate who is carrying a baby for someone else today has no genetic connection to the child. But in the past, a conventional surrogate would use her egg and bear the child for the designated family. Knowing surrogacy success rates can help you comprehend how and why surrogacy is the most effective way to fulfill your family's ambition. This information gives prospective surrogate mothers peace of mind that their time and dedication to supporting a family will almost certainly result in happiness.

Different Surrogacy Arrangements

Surrogacy is seen as a highly delicate and affective matter that profoundly affects all those engaged. Owing to the sensitive nature of surrogacy, it is imperative that all parties involved feel secure and at ease with one another for the procedure to be successful. In terms of surrogacy, many agreements can be made based on the parties' convenience and suitability. As a result, there are now many different types of surrogacy. Every surrogacy agreement is different, and the parties can choose the most suitable and convenient form from a variety of surrogacy arrangement.

Traditional Surrogacy

Also known as "genetic" or "full" surrogacy. Traditionally, the surrogate utilizes her own egg for the surrogate. Using in vitro fertilization (IVF) or artificial insemination, the intended parent's sperm are added to the egg to fertilize it. After giving birth, she gives birth to the child and signs away her parental rights. She bears the child throughout the whole pregnancy. In this instance, the surrogate and the child are biologically connected. Traditional surrogacy can provide unique emotional and legal issues because the surrogate and the child share genetics. Though most states do not provide legal protections for intended parents.

In cases where a surrogate may refuse to give up the child after delivery, many typical surrogacy arrangements have been accomplished without incident. After the baby is delivered, certain state laws compel the surrogate to give up her parental rights; nevertheless, occasionally, surrogates who are biologically related to the child decide otherwise and contest the intended parents' legal claim to the kid. Most surrogacy firms only utilize gestational surrogates because of the lack of legal protection and possibility for issues.

Gestational Surrogacy

This kind of pregnancy involves the implantation of an embryo into the uterus of the surrogate. Using in vitro fertilization (IVF), the embryo is created from the intending parents' egg and sperm or from donors. Since the surrogate did not produce the egg, there is no genetic relationship between the surrogate and the child. If vitro fertilization (IVF) is used to generate the embryo she is carrying, which is subsequently placed into her uterus. The embryo may be formed using biological material from one or both intended parents, or it may be created using donor material, depending on the specifics of the situation. The gestational surrogate goes home until it's time to give birth after being discharged into the care of her preferred OBGYN. Once she becomes pregnant it can be challenging to decide between gestational and traditional surrogacy. To better balance the benefits and drawbacks of each approach, patients should think about the following:

- Can I or my partner provide my surrogate with eggs?

- Do I feel at ease knowing that my baby's biological mother is carrying it?

- What sort of bond do I hope to have with my surrogate?

- Can I afford the expense of gestational surrogacy?

- Is conventional surrogacy legal in my state?

The History of Surrogacy

Despite being as old as the the Scripture, Abraham and Sarah. Attorney Noel Keane arranged the first surrogacy arrangement in law in 1976. It was an uncompensated traditional surrogacy. Following the birth of Louise Brown in 1978, Elizabeth Kane (pseudonym), a traditional surrogate, and her husband arranged the first-ever compensated surrogacy agreement in 1980. Later on, she wrote a book called "Birth Mother," in which she discussed her experiences and regrets.

The well-known Baby M case was one of the most well-known surrogacy situations, and it most likely brought to light the flaws in the traditional surrogacy arrangement. In 1984, Mary Betty Whitehead was employed as a traditional surrogate by Bill and Betty Stern.

After the use of Ms. Whitehead's eggs, the baby was born, and she refused to give up custody, leading to a protracted custody dispute. Ms. Whitehead's parental rights were reinstated after the Supreme Court of New Jersey decided on February 3, 1988, that the surrogacy agreement between the Sterns and her was unlawful. Mr. Bill Stern was given custody, and Ms. Whitehead was given visitation privileges.

The first gestational surrogacy was completed in 1985 during the Baby M case, which set the precedent for future gestational surrogates to be the norm. Avoiding all of the moral and legal dilemmas associated with conventional surrogacy. In another development in year 2014, In a well reported case, an Australian couple recruited a lady who had given birth to twins in 2013 to act as their surrogate mother. A scan performed seven months into the pregnancy revealed she was pregnant with twins, one of whom had Down syndrome.

The surrogate mother refused the intending parents' request for an abortion operation on the afflicted child. The Down syndrome kid was abandoned by the couple after they left with a healthy newborn. When the surrogate mother went public through an Australian charity to gather money for the ailing infant known as infant Gammy, the case gained attention. She not only had Down syndrome, but also had congenital heart issues, which are typically linked to Down syndrome. The response forced Thailand to outlaw paid surrogacy for foreigners and to prohibit surrogate kids from leaving the country with their parents.

A number of celebrities, including Kim Kardashian and Kanye West, have also utilized surrogacy to conceive their own children, May 9, 2019, marked the birth of their last child. The previous child was also born via surrogacy because Kim experienced some serious difficulties during her previous deliveries. Just five months after the birth of their third child, Teigen and John Legend joyfully revealed in 2023 that their fourth kid, Wren Alexander Stephens, had arrived, bringing their family to six members. The 12-time Grammy Award winner confirmed the wonderful news on Instagram on June 28, announcing that their kid was born on June 19, 2023, through surrogacy.

Legal and Ethical Perspective

It has been shown that surrogacy benefits infertile couples. Simultaneously, the growing utilization of this technology has given rise to a number of disputes and contradictory legal matters. These disputes have occasionally exploded into a heated discussion on whether surrogacy is lawful. To comprehend the reasons behind surrogacy, it is vital to have a conversation about this controversy. Furthermore, since the controversy surrounding surrogacy has been brought to light by prominent surrogacy cases worldwide as well as arguments made by legal scholars and commentators.

it is crucial to have this kind of discussion in order to determine how legal systems in other nations should handle surrogacy going forward. The majority of objections to surrogacy are grounded in a variety of moral, ethical, religious, and legal arguments. It is true that morality, ethics, and religious beliefs cannot be completely excluded from a legal discussion. After all, these factors have greatly influenced how cultures see legal matters and have formed the basis of the majority of international legal systems. The idea behind the moral, ethical, and religious arguments against surrogacy is that since God created life, humans shouldn't try to play God by meddling with nature's processes.

The fact that the surrogacy process entails numerous trials using either male or female genetic material or human embryos is another significant concern in this regard. Because some academics believe that human life begins at fertilization, the waste of human embryos is compared to murder. The primary legal challenge to surrogacy targets the fundamental component of the surrogacy process, which is the obligation of a woman to serve as a surrogate. The practice of surrogate and motherhood7 has since drawn a number of criticisms from some academics due to the unacceptable dangers it poses to women, which include psychological, bodily, and symbolic risks like objectification and commercialization.

Legal Procedure

In a typical surrogacy scenario, the woman serving as the surrogate is also the child's biological mother.

States have different regulations when it comes to surrogacy; however, in some cases, further legal action is needed to establish the intended parents as adoptive parents and end the surrogate's parental rights after the child is delivered. Regretfully, this postponement gives the surrogate enough time to decide otherwise after the child is delivered. There have been instances where a surrogate refuse to give up parental rights because they are too devoted to the child.

A drawn-out and expensive legal battle over who is entitled to the child has resulted in many cases. Most intended parents acquire a pre-birth order while the surrogate is pregnant as part of the gestational surrogacy process. A pre-birth order guarantees that the intended parents' names will appear on the baby's birth certificate and legally establishes their rights to the child from the moment of birth. Because the intended parents' legal rights are established prior to the baby's birth and the surrogate cannot subsequently change her mind, this is a crucial step.

Emotional Complications

An attachment will develop between a surrogate and the child she bears. That is quite normal, and when you deal with a respectable organization, they support and counsel surrogates. Because she is biologically related to the child, a conventional surrogate could experience a stronger relationship. Due to their strong emotional connection, she might find it challenging to give the baby to its intended parents after delivery, which would be challenging for all parties. There is no biological bond between a gestational surrogate and the child she bears.

In addition to making the legal requirements of surrogacy simpler, a common reason for women to sign up as gestational surrogates is their desire to give someone else the gift of a child. It's common for them to develop some attachment to the child they carried, but their happiness for assisting another family greatly surpasses the other feelings. One of the main advantages of gestational surrogacy is this.

Although attitudes toward surrogacy have improved and it has become more common, surrogacy is still the most contentious form of assisted reproduction and raises a number of ethical questions. The child is seen as a commodity to be bought and sold, according to many who oppose surrogacy, and some people even consider paying a surrogate to be the same as selling babies.

The possibility of exploitation that arises when economically disadvantaged women bear children for more affluent women is another reason against surrogacy; this is especially evident when the decision to become a surrogate is primarily motivated by financial gain. Procreative liberty is another issue that is brought up by surrogacy: should women be permitted to carry another woman's pregnancy? It's interesting to observe the differences in feminist perspectives on surrogacy: Some believe it to be the ultimate form of female exploitation, while others maintain that women should have control over their reproductive choices and can choose to serve as paid surrogates if they so desire.

Chapter 2

Is Surrogacy Right for You?

Surrogacy is a popular choice for individuals who want to start a family for a variety of reasons, such as infertility, health issues, and male infertility. Miscarriages account for 10–20% of documented pregnancies. When we account for pregnancies that end before a woman misses a menstrual cycle, that number might be as high as 50%. Not every surrogacy journey starts with a diagnosis of infertility. Some people decide on surrogacy for private purposes. For the LGBTQ+ community and single guys, surrogacy is an incredibly popular way to become parents.

Being a surrogate can be a very fulfilling experience. You will create parents, grandparents, aunts, uncles, and cousins, and you will forever alter the lives of family members. Still, being a surrogate involves a lengthy and emotionally taxing process that calls for perseverance and fortitude. Consider carefully if surrogacy is the right decision for you and your family. It is not the correct choice for every woman. If there is no unacceptably high danger to your physical or emotional well-being, you should only agree to be a surrogate.

Surrogate parents choose to become surrogates voluntarily, but parents who conceive through surrogacy typically have no other option. Any pregnancy carries some risk, of course, but no surrogate should put herself at intolerable danger of problems with her physical or mental health. You may be at risk for surrogacy if you are ill, have a history of severe postpartum depression, or experience pregnancy difficulties. Give serious thought to your motivations for wanting to be a surrogate as well as the kind of experience and bond you hope to have with your intended parents.

Being open and truthful about your choices can help you locate the right partner and customize your adventure to suit your needs. For surrogates and their families, surrogacy may be immensely fulfilling, fostering unique relationships between two families and allowing surrogates to demonstrate to their own kids the value of helping others.

Additionally, becoming a surrogate is a huge commitment that will take up a lot of your own time and energy over the course of probably two years. Ensuring that you are aware of the process, ready for the commitment, and that this is the best decision for you and your family is crucial. There are a number of considerations when selecting a surrogate, but the good news is that they are fair. A surrogate need to be able to pass a background investigation and have a history of good pregnancies. Furthermore, surrogates ought to additionally;

- Reside in a state where surrogacy is lawful

- Be in the age range of 21 to 40

- Have a body mass index in the range of 18 to 32

- Possess a history of good reproduction

- Give birth to a healthy child at least once

- Cleared a psychological assessment

- Agree to sign a contract outlining the risks and obligations associated with the pregnancy, prenatal care, and giving up the child after birth

- Accepts medical examinations: Past Events

- HIV and Syphilis screening for infectious disorders

- Screening for genetic diseases: SCD, or genotype

- Rubella vaccination

- Have no drug or alcohol addiction

- Quit smoking and avoid living in a house where there are current smokers

- Hold out on becoming a surrogate for six months after giving delivery

The Right Surrogacy Agency

If you're considering being a surrogate, you should make sure you're dealing with a group of experts who can give you the thorough knowledge, support, and direction you need throughout this momentous occasion.

This is crucial since picking the appropriate surrogacy program will have a major impact. Maybe you've determined that surrogacy is the best option for you. You've done your homework and talked to your family, friends, and doctor. The time has come to select a reliable surrogacy organization. Find out about the standing of several agencies before you begin your investigation. What qualities about them do their website and brand represent? What honors or accolades have they received? Do they follow the American Society for Reproductive Medicine's surrogacy guidelines? It's critical to pay attention to the discourse surrounding an organization and to conduct an in-depth study of the work the agency performs. Start with their requirements for surrogates and screening procedures.

What standards does the organization apply when choosing its surrogates? The caliber of the surrogates and the manner in which an agency handles both intended parents and surrogates are critical factors in a successful surrogacy process. It takes expertise and experience to be a surrogate, so make sure the person you deal with directly has a thorough understanding of the field and the procedure. An efficient surrogacy process requires a lot of resources, so choosing the option that seems to be the cheapest isn't necessarily the best choice.

Instead, you ought to consider how valuable the agency's offerings are. The top surrogacy organizations will go over each expense with you and explain why it is what it is. Openness is crucial. Selecting the ideal surrogacy agency for you and your family is crucial, as there are numerous possibilities available. As a surrogate, you should associate with a company that values and safeguards you. If you're a parent, the proper agency will help you find the ideal surrogate and bring your new family member home.

Selecting the best surrogacy program or agency to support them is one of the largest obstacles intended parents encounter after deciding to use a surrogate to expand their family. Selecting a program, you can completely rely on can make the difference between a stress-filled, successful process and one that is not only professional but also seamless.

Be Aware of the Services Included

Make sure you understand exactly what services are covered by your selected surrogacy agency's program, what services they are unable to assist you with, and the potential cost of any additional services you may require from other crucial service providers before working with them. Some surrogacy firms may not disclose to you up front that they charge a premium for matching services but offer no additional assistance or services at all.

Whether the surrogates have undergone thorough pre-screening before matching is a crucial topic. Certain surrogacy organizations fail to thoroughly vet surrogates prior to placing them with their intended parents. Matches that are not properly and sufficiently screened sometimes end in heartache for all parties involved, as well as wasted time and money. In a similar vein, some agencies might complete all of the pre-screening but fail to make themselves available to you or your surrogate at any point during the procedure.

No matter what comes up, you want to be able to count on your selected agency to help you promptly. Working with a surrogacy agency that provides a comprehensive program and has a team that is not only sensitive and experienced but also really caring and hands-on is ideal. This staff will act as your reliable guide during every stage of the surrogacy journey.

Transparency is Crucial

When using a surrogacy agency, financial transparency is a crucial concern. You're not the only one who finds the price structure of an agency confusing. It might be difficult for intended parents to figure out exactly what each service offers and how much they will charge throughout the surrogacy process. In order to feel well-represented in the long run and to make an informed decision, it is imperative that you have reliable information.

You should be able to find and compare the actual costs for each agency if you delve into the pricing and ask specific questions about what is included in the estimated costs and fees for the surrogate. It is a red flag that you shouldn't think about collaborating with a certain agency if it is difficult to obtain this information.

Is There A Past?

Does the surrogacy agency you're thinking about have a history of fulfilling matches? For what duration has it been operating? What position do they hold in the sector? What level of involvement do they have in assisted reproduction? Experience is quite valuable. Select a family-building program and staff that have the necessary training and years of expertise.

Which medical and psychological screening methods does a certain agency employ to evaluate possible surrogates? Have they actually met them in person? Do they run criminal and background checks? To what extent are they selective? Do they use other sources or hire their own surrogates? Intended parents will receive this information from a reputable, lawful surrogacy agency, and most importantly, they will be made fully aware of the procedure.

Recognize the Limitations of "Screening"

Most organizations just go through a paper review of the potential gestational surrogate. Before matching, they don't thoroughly screen their applications. You may waste time and money if your fertility facility rejects the surrogate after matching them if a thorough pre-screening wasn't completed before matching. The assurance that everything will go smoothly and that you can continue to develop a relationship with the surrogate after initial screening is provided. Proper pre-screening entails:

- A home visit from a social worker when necessary

- An in-person psychological evaluation for the surrogate, her spouse, or other significant other. An insurance review to see whether the surrogate is covered for pregnancy and delivery

- Assistance in securing suitable health insurance coverage

- Financial evaluation of the surrogate's household income and financial stability

- Medical clearance from the surrogate's OB

- Criminal and civil background checks for the surrogate and spouse or significant other

For this reason, it is crucial that you select your reproductive endocrinologist (RE) before the match. Each medical facility sets its own requirements and standards for qualified gestational surrogates. It is essential that your own RE has the chance to evaluate records before an official match in order to match you with a surrogate appropriately and prevent any problems down the road.

What About Lawsuits?

Has the surrogacy agency been sued by intended parents or surrogates in the past? In that case, how have these legal disputes been settled? Although a lawsuit doesn't always indicate incompetence, it can provide insight into the professionalism of the agency. You must be confident that the agency you have selected is a good fit before you can proceed. One who can assist you through every stage, from starting to being a being a baby, and provide answers to all of your questions.

Budgeting and Financial Planning

A lot of prospective parents believe that having a child is an incredibly valuable experience. Naturally, the truth is that establishing a family always comes with expenses. That cost might easily reach the six figures when using surrogacy to become a parent. Inflation has driven up the cost of surrogacy during the past year, as it has many other expenses. The precise cost of using a surrogate to carry a child will differ for every family and be influenced by a number of variables, including insurance coverage, the location of the parents and surrogate, and the outcome of in vitro fertilization. The entire expenditure may vary between $225,000 and $100,000.

Cost Breakdown

The cost of surrogacy is composed of multiple factors:

Embryo Formation: Prior to choosing surrogacy, many couples had already collaborated with a fertility clinic to create embryos. Range of costs: $20,000 to $50,000.

Donating Eggs: Paying for a donor egg may also be necessary for some heterosexual couples as well as same sex couples. Range of costs: $20,000 to $30,000.

Costs Associated with Agencies: The scope of an agency's services can have a big impact on the cost. While some organizations offer legal services and medical screening as part of their package, others do not. I strongly advise prospective parents to search for the agency that best suits their needs and to weigh the costs in relation to the services the agency provides in exchange. Price range: up to $30,000.

Legal Fees: It's crucial to deal with a lawyer who can draft the required documentation outlining the compensation system and what will happen in the event of pregnancy difficulties if the agency does not provide legal assistance. You might also require assistance with adoption and pre- or post-birth legal documentation. Range of costs: $7,000 to $15,000.

Basic Compensation: This is the money that your family directly pays the surrogate for carrying and giving birth to the child on your behalf. The surrogate's location and prior experience serving as a surrogate will determine this price. Range of costs: $30,000 to $70,000.

Contingent Surrogacy Fees: Should issues emerge during the pregnancy which can include anything from unexpected twins (in the event that an embryo splits) to an unforeseen C-section the intended family may be required to pay these additional payments. Range of costs: $15,000 to $30,000.

Insurance: While intended families pay the premiums and deductibles for their surrogate's insurance plan while they are working together, most regular health insurance plans do not cover surrogate pregnancies. A few insurance policies also include additional coverage for pregnancy and delivery, which intended families can purchase on behalf of their surrogates. Range of costs: $12,000 to $30,000.

Additional Costs: Intended families should consider a number of other, lesser costs while evaluating the cost of surrogacy.

These include maternity supplies (clothing and prenatal care), as well as travel if the gestational carrier is not local. In the meantime, expectant parents should start preparing their supply of cribs, bottles, and diapers, among other necessities that they will require right away following the birth. Price range: not fixed.

Payment Options for Gestational Surrogacy

Considering how expensive gestational surrogacy can be, it's critical to have a financial plan in place for when the time comes. That strategy will probably involve a mix of the following:

Benefits Offered at Work: Employers rarely include surrogacy insurance in their benefit packages, but in 2022, 15% did, and by 2024, 19% were thinking about doing so.

Health Coverage: The expenses of a surrogate pregnancy are typically not covered by health insurance plans; however, many do cover some of the costs of operations needed for intended parents. In the event that your carrier does not reside in your state, you may want to think about how your plan handles out-of-network physicians, as health insurance will also cover the baby's postpartum costs.

Individual Funds: If you anticipate that your family's history may involve a surrogacy, even modest monthly contributions to a special account might build up over time. It can take up to 18 months to find a donor; therefore, you can carry on with this procedure even after you start working with an agency.

Support from Friends Or Relatives: In order to help pay for the surrogacy, intended parents frequently turn to their friends and family.

Awards: Certain organizations offer financial assistance to couples who are experiencing infertility. While some of these subsidies are intended to cover IVF treatments, others may be used to cover surrogacy-specific expenses.

Chapter 3

Medical Procedure and Reproductive Technology

In vitro fertilization (IVF) is the process by which the surrogate becomes pregnant in a gestational surrogacy. The surrogate will not be genetically connected to the child, instead, an embryo will be generated in a lab and put in her uterus. Four stages of the IVF procedure for gestational carriers are explained below. Firstly, you will go through a medical exam to make sure you are healthy enough to carry a surrogate pregnancy before starting the medical surrogacy process.

You will also receive a routine physical examination, blood testing, and an ultrasound to look at your uterus. In order to screen for infectious diseases, your partner or spouse might also need to have blood work completed. To control your cycle, the doctor could prescribe hormones and birth control tablets. This allows the doctor to monitor your cycle more closely and guarantees that you are prepared to receive the embryos at the precise moment.

You will probably be getting estrogen replacements and progesterone injections at this stage of the surrogacy procedure to help keep your hormone levels constant and support a stable pregnancy. Up until the 12th week of pregnancy, when the placenta usually takes over hormone synthesis, you will continue to take these hormones. When the embryos have grown for five days and you are five days past mid-cycle, the embryo transfer operation will take place.

A catheter that is placed into the uterus through the cervix will be used to transfer the embryo or embryos. You won't be sedated throughout the relatively short and painless process. After the embryo transfer, you might need to take a few days off from activity. You will go back to the fertility clinic around a week following the embryo transfer so the doctor can check your levels of pregnancy hormones. A positive, stable pregnancy is indicated by an HCG value of 50 or above; multiple pregnancies may be indicated by a count of more than 200.

A few days later, the doctors will perform another HCG test to make sure that these levels are rising; they should double every two days. It's crucial to keep in mind that getting a surrogate pregnant can require more than one embryo transfer. Throughout this process, you will be attentively observed. Finish the ultrasound after six weeks and start prenatal care. Around the sixth week of pregnancy, the doctor will do an ultrasound following a successful embryo transfer. You might be sent to see your own OB/GYN if a heartbeat is seen during the ultrasound, or you might get another ultrasound about a month before leaving the fertility clinic's office and seeing your own OB/GYN. You will receive prenatal care at this stage of the process, just like you would with any other pregnancy.

Understanding the IVF Process

In vitro fertilization is referred to as IVF. It's among the forms of assisted reproductive technology (ART) that are more known. IVF is chosen by individuals for a variety of reasons, such as infertility problems or a partner's pre-existing medical condition. If they are older mothers or if other reproductive treatments have not worked for them, some will consider in vitro fertilization (IVF). IVF is an additional reproductive option for individuals who want to have a family on their own or for same-sex couples. One possibility for IVF is if you or your partner have;

- Fallopian tubes are broken or obstructed

- Endometriosis

- Sperm issues or low count

- Other ovarian problems, such as polycystic ovary syndrome (PCOS),

- Fibroids in uterus

- Issues relating to your uterus

- Risk of inheriting a disease

- Unknown cause of infertility

- Are making use of gestational surrogates or egg donors.

In order to help the sperm, fertilize an egg and aid the fertilized egg's implantation in your uterus, in vitro fertilization (IVF) employs a combination of medications and surgical techniques. You start by taking medicine, which ages some of your eggs and prepares them for fertilization. After that, the doctor removes the eggs from your body and fertilizes them in a lab by combining them with sperm. Then they insert one or more embryos, which are fertilized eggs, straight into your uterus. If some of the embryos implant in the lining of your uterus, pregnancy will result. Although many people require more than one round of IVF to become pregnant, it can occasionally work on the first try. If you're suffering fertility issues, IVF will undoubtedly enhance your chances of getting pregnant, but there's no assurance as every person's body is unique and IVF won't be effective for everyone.

Stages of IVF Treatment

The steps involved in IVF are as follows:

Day 1: Estrogen or Birth Control Pills

Your doctor can recommend estrogen or birth control tablets prior to the start of IVF treatment. This is used to regulate the timing of your menstrual cycle and prevent the formation of ovarian cysts. During the egg retrieval process, it enables your healthcare professional to manage your care and get the most developed eggs possible.

Day 2 - 4: Stimulation of The Ovaries

Every month, a batch of eggs starts to grow throughout a healthy person of reproductive age's natural cycle. Usually, only one egg reaches the maturity required for ovulation. The rest of the immature eggs in that group break apart. You will administer injectable hormone drugs during your IVF cycle in order to promote the full and simultaneous maturation of all the eggs in that cycle. This implies that you might have multiple eggs as opposed to just one, as in a natural cycle. Your medical history, age, AMH (anti-Mullerian hormone) level, and past IVF cycle response to ovarian stimulation will all be taken into account when determining the kind, dosage, and frequency of prescription drugs.

Day 5-7: Monitoring

Blood hormone levels and ultrasounds are used to track how your ovaries are responding to the medicine. For two weeks, monitoring can take place every day or every few days. The majority of stimulations last eight to fourteen days. Healthcare professionals utilize ultrasound to examine your ovaries and uterus during monitoring visits. The eggs are too tiny for ultrasonography. However, your medical professionals will count and measure the ovarian follicles that are developing. Your ovaries have tiny sacs called follicles that are meant to hold a single egg. Each follicle's size reveals how mature the egg inside of it is. A developed egg is present in the majority of follicles that are larger than 14 mm. Less than 14-mm follicles are more likely to contain immature eggs that won't fertilize.

Day 8–10: Trigger shot

A "trigger shot" is administered to complete the maturation of your eggs in preparation for egg retrieval when they are ready for it (as indicated by your ultrasound and hormone levels). The trigger injection should be given precisely 36 hours prior to the time you have set for egg retrieval.

Day 11–12: Egg Retrieval

Your doctor inserts a thin needle into each of your ovaries through your vagina, using an ultrasound to guide the needle. Your eggs are extracted from each follicle using a suction device that is attached to the needle. Your eggs are put on a plate with a unique solution on it. Next, the dish is placed in a controlled environment—an incubator. In order to minimize discomfort during this treatment, medication and moderate anesthesia are employed. The "trigger shot," or last hormone injection, is given 36 hours prior to egg retrieval.

Day 13–14: Fertilization

The embryologist will attempt to use intracytoplasmic sperm injection, or ICSI, to fertilize all mature eggs the afternoon after your egg retrieval surgery. This implies that each developed egg will receive an injection of sperm. You cannot do ICSI on immature eggs. The developing eggs will be put in a dish with nourishment and sperm.

Seldom do immature eggs complete their development in the dish. The sperm in the dish can then try to fertilize the egg if the immature one does not break through. Seventy percent of mature eggs will fertilize on average. For instance, roughly seven of the ten mature eggs that are recovered will fertilize. The fertilized egg will develop into an embryo if all goes well. It is possible to freeze some eggs prior to fertilization for later use if there are an unusually high number of eggs or if you decide not to fertilize all of them.

Day 15–19: Development of The Embryo

We will be closely monitoring the development of your embryos over the next five to six days. For your embryo to be ready for transfer into your uterus, it must overcome several obstacles. 50% of fertilized embryos reach the blastocyst stage on average. The stage is ideal for transferring to your uterus. For instance, three or four of the seven fertilized eggs can reach the blastocyst stage of development. Usually, the remaining 50% are thrown after failing to advance. On the fifth or sixth day after fertilization, all viable embryos will be preserved andused for subsequent embryo transfers.

Day 20–21: Transfer of Embryos

Fresh embryo transfers and frozen embryo transfers are the two types of embryo transfers. Your doctor can talk to you about using fresh or frozen embryos and determine which is best for you given your particular circumstances. The identical transfer procedure is used for transfers of both fresh and frozen embryos. The name itself suggests the primary distinction. If you have a fresh embryo transfer, your embryo will be placed in your uterus three to seven days following the egg retrieval process.

This embryo is "fresh," meaning it hasn't been frozen. Frozen embryos (from a prior IVF cycle or donor eggs) are thawed and put into your uterus during a frozen embryo transfer. Due to practical considerations and the higher likelihood of a live birth, this is a more widely used procedure. Transfers of frozen embryos can happen years after fertilization and egg retrieval. You will take oral, injectable, vaginal, or transdermal hormones as part of the initial phase of a frozen embryo transfer to get your uterus ready to accept an embryo.

This often entails taking medication orally for 14–21 days, then receiving injections for 6 days. During this time, you will usually have two or three appointments to have a blood test to determine your hormone levels and an ultrasound to check the readiness of your uterus. You will be given an appointment for the embryo transfer process when your uterus is prepared. If you're using fresh embryos, the procedure is similar, but the embryos are transferred three to five days after they are harvested.

It is a straightforward process that doesn't involve anesthesia: embryo transfer. It feels like a pap smear or pelvic exam. A tiny catheter is passed through the cervix and into the uterus, and a speculum is positioned into the vagina. One or more embryos are contained in a syringe that is fastened to the other end of the catheter. Using a catheter, the embryos are inserted into the uterus. Usually, the process takes less than ten minutes.

Day 22–30: Conception

When the embryo inserts itself into the lining of your uterus, pregnancy results. In the nine to fourteen days following embryo transfer, your healthcare professional will conduct a blood test to assess whether or not you are pregnant. The same steps apply to donor eggs. The egg donor will finish the egg retrieval and ovarian stimulation processes. Following fertilization, the embryo is transferred to the intended parent (either with or without different types of fertility drugs). 7It's crucial to keep in mind that every individual's experience with IVF can be different and that getting pregnant might require more than one cycle. Mood changes, bruising from shots, bleeding, infection, cramps, bloating, breast tenderness, headaches, and adverse reactions to medications are modest symptoms that can be experienced following an embryo transfer.

Anticipated Difficulties in IVF Process

Multiple pregnancies: This is one of the most frequent IVF side effects. There is a greater likelihood of many embryos implanting in the uterus, which could result in the delivery of twins, triplets, or even more. Premature labor and low birth weight in kids are two issues during pregnancy and childbirth that can be made more likely by multiple pregnancies.

Ovarian Hyperstimulation Syndrome (OHSS): When a woman's ovaries are stimulated to create many eggs during the IVF procedure, OHSS, a potentially dangerous complication, may arise. Abdominal pain, bloating, nausea, and vomiting are some possible symptoms. In extreme situations, OHSS can result in renal failure or blood clots, as well as fluid accumulation in the chest and belly.

Ectopic Pregnancy: Usually in one of the fallopian tubes, ectopic pregnancy is the result of a fertilized egg implanting outside of the uterus. This can be a potentially fatal illness that needs immediate medical attention. Women with a history of pelvic inflammatory illness or those who have undergone prior pelvic operations, such as tubal ligation, are more susceptible to ectopic pregnancy.

IVF Rounds That Fail: IVF is not always successful, and some couples may need to try several times before getting pregnant. IVF cycle failures can have a variety of causes, such as poor embryo quality, unsuccessful implantation, or underlying illnesses that impair fertility.

Emotional Stress: IVF can be an intellectually and emotionally draining procedure for couples. One's mental health may suffer as a result of the operations' stress, the cost involved, and the uncertainty around the results. During the IVF process, it's critical for couples to have a solid support network and to think about getting counseling or therapy.

Financial Burden: The cost of IVF therapy can be high, and many insurance policies do not cover it. Couples may have to cover their own costs for prescription drugs, medical procedures, and other associated costs. The psychological and financial hardship of the IVF procedure may be exacerbated. To sum up, for infertile couples, in vitro fertilization (IVF) can be a successful reproductive treatment.

It is not without possible complications, though. Before choosing a course of treatment, couples should talk to their healthcare physician about the advantages and disadvantages of IVF and weigh all of their alternatives. To improve your chances of success, make sure you closely adhere to the following guidelines:

Keep Up a Healthy Lifestyle: Living a healthy lifestyle can increase fertility and increase the likelihood that IVF will be successful. This entails controlling stress, exercising frequently, and obtaining adequate sleep.

Adhere to The Directions on Your Medication: During IVF, you will probably be prescribed a number of drugs. Take these drugs exactly as prescribed by your physician.

Keep All of Your Doctor's Appointments: IVF requires several visits. It is critical that you show up for all of these appointments so that your doctor can assess your progress and modify your treatment plan as needed.

What Not to Do During IVF

The first thing you should never do when undergoing IVF is smoke or drink. These behaviors can have a detrimental effect on both your fertility and the outcome of the procedure. It's advisable to stay away from these things completely. Avoid intense exercise. Although exercise is vital, intense exercise might overwork your body and may affect your ability to conceive. Limit your exercise to mild forms like yoga or walking. Don't miss meals. Eating a balanced, healthy diet is crucial during in vitro fertilization. Missing meals might upset your body's equilibrium and have a detrimental effect on your chances of succeeding.

Is IVF Painful?

The discomfort and suffering associated with in vitro fertilization (IVF) can differ from person to person. The following are some things that could hurt or cause discomfort during an IVF cycle:

Hormone Injections: The purpose of hormone injections is to encourage the ovaries to generate a large number of eggs. At the injection site, some women may feel pain, swelling, and bruises.

Egg Retrieval: To remove the eggs from the ovaries, a tiny surgical incision is made in the vaginal wall using a needle. Since you will be sedated during this process, you shouldn't experience any pain.

Embryo Transfer: This technique entails putting fertilized embryos inside the uterus. Although this surgery is normally painless, some women may feel a little discomfort or cramps. It's crucial to remember that IVF-related pain and discomfort are typically minor and transient. To help you manage any pain or discomfort you may encounter, your doctor might prescribe medication and other measures.

Donation of Sperm and Eggs

Egg donation, sperm donation, and surrogacy are attractive choices for many infertile individuals to expand their family. These options may not be exactly the route you had anticipated taking, but they can have excellent success rates, and patients who select them often express great satisfaction in making that decision. It might be difficult to hear that using donor eggs or sperm is your greatest chance of becoming a parent, and most people react strongly to this news.

For many people, a biological connection is highly important, and it might be difficult to accept that this is not feasible. The majority of our patients who use donor eggs or sperm tell us that the pregnancy experience provides a tremendous intimacy and connection with the baby every flutter and kick increase your bond—although everyone responds differently. You will go through the labor and delivery procedure, hold your newborn initially, and then cohabit and live with the child you brought into the world.

Egg Donation

Despite the fact that every woman of legal age is eligible to donate eggs, egg donors must fulfill a number of requirements, and only a tiny number are chosen out of every 100 applications. In actuality, less than 1% of applicants are accepted by many banks and donor organizations. Among the requirements for donors are good health and a clean medical record.

Additionally, donors must pass genetic, physical, and psychological tests. Furthermore, substance abuse and other high-risk activities are prohibited. And these are only a few of the safety measures implemented to guarantee that the donors possess healthy, viable eggs. Of course, decisions about accepting a donor are not just based on medical considerations.

For instance, a person's race, ethnicity, or physical characteristics may be relevant. There will be a difference in the demand for different minorities. Another important factor in the application process is education. It is preferred to have an egg donor with a degree from an elite university, such as an Ivy League school. Giving a family the resources, they need to succeed is a powerful incentive for many egg donors. Some egg donors feel compelled to give back and make a contribution that will benefit future families because of their personal experiences with friends or family who have previously used egg donors.

Others wish to make it possible for same-sex couples to start families biologically in a way that they might not be able to in any other case. For some, receiving payment influences their choice to donate. Although it varies, the remuneration is often in the range of $10,000. Because egg donation is a tough process, compensation plays a significant role in the process. Prior to the extraction date, egg donors must undergo fertility treatments, take daily injections to stimulate their ovaries, and collaborate closely with a physician who closely monitors their health. After that, while they are sedated, they must endure a process to have their eggs removed.

Donation of Sperm

Although sperm donation is far less difficult than egg donation, the selection procedure for sperm donors can be just as competitive. Sperm donation receives far more applications than egg donation, yet only a very small portion of candidates are chosen to give. It's imperative that sperm donors have no medical history or substance misuse history. Highly educated sperm donors are preferred, just like egg donors. Aside from that, factors like physical characteristics and ethnic origin are also considered.

While choosing a donor, many parents take into account factors such as having a comparable height or hair color to one of the parents or having the same racial background because they value these relationships with their future child. To be eligible, applicants must also have a healthy and high count of sperm. The donor's samples will be screened by sperm banks to see if they are of sufficient quality.

Sperm donors are paid as well, but they receive significantly less than egg donors; if they contribute numerous times a month, they typically receive $1,000 or more in compensation. Most sperm donors feel the same way about egg donors. Most are concerned with assisting same-sex or infertile couples in starting families and hope that their assistance will one day transform their life and grant them the much-desired child. Donors of both eggs and sperm donate a portion of themselves to enable families to create the lives of their dreams. They are aware that people who go through the effort of looking for and using their donations are sincerely hoping to become parents.

How to Become an Identified Donor?

It's likely that intended parents may look through anonymous donor profiles before looking for an egg or sperm donation. These profiles may contain images of the donor as a baby in addition to standard, non-identifying details on the donor's history and looks. Whether the donor wants to remain anonymous or to be identified is frequently mentioned in these profiles. You probably won't get any more personal information about an anonymous contributor than what is listed on their page if you decide to collaborate with them.

In a similar vein, neither you nor your child's information will be sent to the donor. Non-anonymous donors, also referred to as named or known donors, might nevertheless be prepared to offer identifying details, establish communication with the intended parents, and accept data regarding the intended parents and their offspring. Many donation programs retain this personal data and grant access to the donor-conceived child upon reaching the age of 18.

Why Choose a Non-Anonymous Donor?

One can draw a comparison between the bond between an adopted child and their biological family and that between a child conceived through donor sperm or egg. The rise in open adoption agreements has made it abundantly evident that understanding one's genetic background can have a significant impact on identity formation, self-assurance, and other aspects of life. Children conceived by donation have the same rights. There are numerous advantages to looking for an identifiable donor, even though it could seem easier to select an anonymous sperm or egg donor.

The following are some of the main arguments in favor of using an openly identifiable sperm or egg donor:

Family medical history: Although it is frozen in time, you will receive a good deal of information about the health history of your egg or sperm donor's family. You can inquire about any recent medical advancements in the donor's family if your child subsequently develops a medical problem and your donor is publicly disclosed. In order to provide intended parents with constant access to the most recent medical and health information for their children, identified donors establish a lifeline.

Siblings and genetic ties: Offspring conceived through donor conception may have a large number of half-siblings and even more cousins. Donor-conceived individuals do not need to worry about their genetic links if they may directly find out about their half siblings through the Donor Sibling Registry or through direct communication with their donor.

Sense of identity: All kids are curious about their origins and identities. These might be tough questions to respond to for kids born from anonymous sperm or egg donations.

Implantation and Embryo Transfer

The final step in the in vitro fertilization process is embryo transfer. It is an extremely crucial process. Even with an excellent IVF laboratory culture environment, a poorly executed embryo transfer by the doctor can spoil the whole affair. The meticulous positioning of the embryos at the appropriate site close to the center of the endometrial cavity, with the least amount of damage and manipulation, is essential to the success of the entire IVF cycle.

An embryo generated through in vitro fertilization (IVF) is put into the uterus of a gestational carrier (surrogate) during a medical procedure known as surrogate embryo transfer. In order to increase the likelihood of a successful implantation and pregnancy, the embryos which are usually generated using the genetic material of the intended parents or donors are carefully chosen for transfer.

With the help of a gestational carrier, people or couples who are unable to carry a pregnancy themselves can have a biological tie to their child through the process of embryo transfer to a surrogate mother. All that is needed for the embryo transfer procedure are the highest-caliber medical staff and a carefully thought-out treatment plan that is tailored to each intended parent's unique situation. The key processes involved in transferring an embryo to a surrogate are as follows:

Preparation: To make sure they are suitable for the process, the intended parents and gestational carrier may go through medical examinations and screenings prior to the transfer. Medication is used to get the gestational carrier ready for implantation.

Embryo Selection: Using their own genetic material or that of a sperm or egg donor. The intended parents may have previously conducted in vitro fertilization (IVF) to develop embryos. The most viable and healthy embryos are chosen for transfer, improving the likelihood that the resulting child will have the highest possible health.

Transfer Process: An outpatient, less invasive process, an embryo transfer, is usually performed. A tube containing the chosen embryos is gently placed into the uterus of the gestational carrier. After this, the embryos are discharged into the uterus.

Post-Transfer Care: The gestational carrier may be recommended to rest and abstain from vigorous activity for a specific amount of time following the transfer.

Pregnancy Testing: To ascertain whether the surgery was effective, a pregnancy test is performed 10–14 days following the transfer. The intended parents excitedly await the growth and development of their unborn child, while the gestational carrier continues to get prenatal treatment if the test yields a good result. In the event that the pregnancy test is negative, the intended parents may choose to use the same surrogate going forward or look into alternative surrogate choices until they get the desired positive outcome.

Stages of Embryo development

The initial stage of the development of an embryo is fertilization, and the blastocyst stage is the final. The key phases of embryonic development are as follows:

Fertilization: The sperm enters the egg during this phase and fertilizes it.

Two Cell Stage: The fertilized egg divides into two cells during the two-cell stage.

Four Cell Stage: Four-cell stage: Two cells divide further to become four cells.

Morula Stage: During this phase, cells start to group together and form.

Chapter 4

Pregnancy and Beyond

Surrogate birthing entails special emotions, difficulties, and health issues. Despite the complexity of the process, many surrogates report feeling happy and purposeful. This may give you comfort. Research on the effects of surrogacy on the person carrying the pregnancy, the children born through surrogacy, and the people who will parent the kid is still lacking significantly. Your physical and mental well-being are crucial as a surrogate. Throughout this process, there are things you can do to take care of your entire self. This post will explain what surrogacy is and what happens to a surrogate after delivering birth.

Supporting Your Surrogate During Pregnancy

Although becoming a surrogate is a wonderful gift, the hundreds of women who choose to undertake this path each year may face some particular difficulties. For the surrogate, her family, and the couple for whom she is carrying the pregnancy, it is an extremely delicate moment. Although women choose to become surrogates for a variety of reasons, they will all require additional support and assistance during the pregnancy.

Being pregnant is a big event in and of itself, but bearing a pregnancy for someone else is truly amazing. There are many things you can do to support your surrogate during her pregnancy, whether you are the parents working with a gestational carrier or perhaps someone you know and love is carrying a pregnancy for another.

Cleaning Duties

This is a top choice for both surrogates and expectant mothers. Being pregnant is a physically difficult time! Pregnant women find housework and tasks difficult, from morning sickness to figuring out how to reach the sink to clean dishes over a growing belly. Even if they don't live with their surrogate, parents can still be a great assistance with chores. Setting up a housekeeper to come once every two weeks can be very beneficial as it relieves the burden on the homeowner and her spouse.

Serve Meals

Taking the evening off from cooking is a very kind gesture. To save her from having to prepare or clean up afterward, ask for her favorite restaurant or site to have food delivered.

Aid Her in Unwinding

Like every pregnancy, surrogacy has its share of discomforts and may be extremely taxing on the body.

It's crucial to support your surrogate in maintaining their composure and comfort! This isn't limited to partners or close relatives. Send your surrogate for a spa day if you are the intended parent, or locate a massage parlor in your community that provides a pregnancy package so she may go on a regular basis.

Give her a gift certificate for prenatal yoga sessions if the doctor approves and she's an active maternity patient. Prenatal yoga can be calming and helpful throughout labor and delivery. You will know that she will appreciate you going above and beyond to make her pregnancy as comfortable as possible.

Spend Time With Each Other

Take some time to get to know your surrogate better! Take her out to dinner or just have a conversation over a cup of coffee (or tea!). Getting to know one another better might aid in facilitating communication during this process, particularly given how emotionally intense it is.

Check in With Her

It can be challenging to end a pregnancy, particularly for a surrogate! Apart from the typical pregnancy discomforts, she probably worries about the delivery, the changes that will occur, and the experience of returning the baby to its parents.

If you are the intended parent, check in with her from time to time to see how she's doing and if she needs anything. It's crucial to avoid doing this too frequently, since some women may feel as though they are being micromanaged. Early in the relationship, it could be beneficial to talk about what you both think is appropriate and what you expect from each other.

Question Her

Ask her if you're unsure! Find out what she needs to ease into the pregnancy or to be more comfortable. Occasionally, this might simply entail additional assistance around the house, or it could indicate something worse. once a week. You may help your surrogate tremendously throughout her pregnancy.

Preparing for Birth and Delivery

Is the time now? The water in your surrogate has broken. The frequency and intensity of her contractions are growing. She's prepared. The time has come- the one you have been anticipating. Depending on how it is delivered, planned or unplanned, vaginal or via C-section?. By the time of birth, you will receive notification to come to the hospital. If you have remained emotionally close to your surrogate throughout the pregnancy, they may contact you personally or through your case consultant. It's crucial for surrogates and IPs, as well as IPs and the hospital, to communicate.

Talk about the circumstances with the floor supervisor well in advance, and let them know about the post-birth routine that you and your surrogate have decided upon. The identity of the parents should be emphasized the most. Be aware of the procedures for giving birth, recovering from it, nursing, cutting the cord, etc. Considering how hectic the day will be, it's crucial to go over each stage of the procedure to prevent confusion.

On the Way to The Medical Facility

Please remember this above all else, just like you would for any expectant couple: drive carefully. Even if you and your partner are not in labor, you and your partner will probably be quite excited and nervous, which will raise your adrenaline levels. Have patience? You'll succeed in getting there. Like any other expecting couple, make sure to include a baby bag. Allow your substitute to sleep with a transitional object that will carry her aroma. The surrogate's aroma will naturally reassure the infant.

On Arrival

In a perfect world, you and your surrogate would arrive at the same time. This will facilitate the hospital staff's ability to identify you all as a single, coherent unit. The IPs and surrogates, however, frequently arrive at various times.

Should you have maintained contact with the medical professionals, they will be prepared for your arrival. Like any other patient, you will check in and, if a room is available, be assigned to your own room. You will be allowed to enter the delivery room to give birth if your surrogate consents.

During Labor and Delivery

It's ultimately up to your surrogate whether or not you'll be in the delivery room, no matter how close you are to her. Unless the surrogate specifically asks them to be there, the intended parents are not permitted in the delivery room. This relates only to their capacity to provide a calm, concentrated birthing environment for your child. In the event that your surrogate has a C-section, keep in mind that, because of space constraints, most operating rooms can only accommodate one more person.

Once more, the surrogate decides who that one person will be. What will happen when you and your surrogate decide to sever the cord once more? After a brief assessment to confirm the baby's health, you will be able to hold your child for a few minutes at the very least. Eventually, the infant will be taken to the obstetrics room for a more in-depth assessment.

Outside the Delivery Room

If you aren't there when your child is born, you'll probably be kept informed about the labor progress as you wait in a nearby room. Following delivery, the infant will have a brief inspection before being taken straight to the parents for a first glance at their new kid. Like with an in-room delivery, the infant is taken back to the obstetrics room for a more detailed examination.

Should you have executed a pre-birth order, the hospital will immediately award you complete guardianship. Together, you can decide if you want your surrogate to spend time with the newborn after delivery to ease their adjustment into the real world. Providing the IPs with the Gift of Life. A few hours after birth, the surrogate, infant, and IPs will probably be brought to the recovery unit at the same time.

This allows the surrogate to relax and recuperate while also providing IPs with a chance to form a bond with their child. It's impossible to describe the feeling you have when your surrogate gives you your child in person. As a symbolic gesture, some surrogates particularly request that the nurses be the ones to give you your child. It's a breathtaking love for the baby you've worked so hard for and the lady who gave birth to you, but it can also be extremely stressful emotionally.

Postpartum Care

When the surrogate and the kid are both physically ready, the baby will be handed to the IPs. It is extremely recommended that the infant and IP have skin to skin contact. This will strengthen the physical relationship between you and your baby while also boosting his immune system. As soon as feasible after delivery, make sure to optimize physical comfort. And last, if you want to keep up this amazing relationship that has allowed you to grow your family, it's critical that you continue to see your surrogate after giving birth. Give her some flowers. Say "thank you." Continue to support your surrogate. She still needs to spend weeks recovering from giving birth, while you have been given the amazing gift of life.

Transition to Parenthood

It will feel like the much-awaited finish line of the marathon that is the surrogacy procedure when your kid is finally brought home. Although your surrogacy journey and your family are now complete, your surrogacy story will carry on long after the procedural formalities are completed.

Your Parenting Journey

You could be concerned about your own well-being as an intended parent (IP) following the surrogacy procedure. Preparing for a newborn is a significant task. Like any pregnant parent, you will probably become increasingly nervous about parenting as the baby's due date approaches, especially if this is your first child. Even though every parent's experience is unique, there are some tried-and-true parenting tips that might be useful. Take the suggestions that appeal to you and disregard the rest; don't feel pressured to implement them all!

Breastfeeding After Surrogacy

Speaking with her doctor is the first step for any soon-to-be mother who wants to breastfeed. It will be especially crucial to cooperate with your doctor as you start and stop using drugs to encourage lactation if you plan to nurse your surrogate child. Nursing a surrogate baby is similar to nursing any other newborn, although it does require some preliminary planning. Your doctor may prescribe hormones (typically birth control tablets) months before your child is born. Your body is tricked by these hormones into believing you are pregnant, which is the precursor to the creation of milk. Use drugs and supplements to replace the hormones.

Your doctor will advise stopping the birth control pill before the baby is born and may prescribe herbal supplements and drugs that aid in increasing milk production. Get your pump going. Stopping the hormones and starting milk-producing drugs will also cause you to start pumping, progressively increasing the amount of time and how often you do it until you start making milk.

When you get ready for the birth of your child, your supply should progressively rise in accordance with your doctor's recommendations and induced lactation protocols. Begin nursing while adding to your milk supply. Even though lactation can be induced, most women are unable to make enough milk on their own to meet the needs of a newborn.

As an alternative, supplemental nursing systems (SNSs) are often used by intended moms to make sure their infants are receiving enough nutrition. Just fill the SNS container with supplemental milk (donated breastmilk, surrogate's breastmilk, milk you've already pumped, or formula) and secure the tubes to your chest. Your baby will receive both the milk from the SNS and any milk you are generating when you nurse him or her with the SNS. This ensures your baby eats lots of food and helps him or her become comfortable to nursing.

It's critical to keep in mind that every mother has a unique nursing experience, and your level of success may differ depending on several variables. Whether or not the child is surrogate-born, not everyone is a good fit for breastfeeding, particularly when it involves induced lactation. Consider what she needs, or simply ask her how you can assist. Talking with your surrogate coordinator might also help you come up with ideas if you're an intended parent. A successful journey depends on your support as well as the support of those in her immediate vicinity.

Breastfeeding as A Surrogate

Utilizing the surrogate's breastmilk is an additional choice for intended parents who are ardent supporters of nursing. After the baby is born, a lot of surrogates are ready to keep pumping for up to six weeks. Regardless of whether the intended mother chooses to breastfeed or not, this milk can be used to feed the baby through a bottle or an additional nursing system. While it is not necessary for surrogates to pump, those who do so invest a significant amount of time and effort into pumping and sending the milk to the intended family. You will soon learn how difficult pumping can be if you or your spouse decide to induce lactation.

Comparably, if your surrogate consents to pump for you, she will have to do it frequently even at night which might be inconvenient and demand a significant commitment of time. Surrogates should be paid for their prolonged dedication to the intended family because of these reasons. The majority of agencies recommend $200–$250 in pumping per week, which includes all shipping expenses and process-related consumables. Prior to the embryo transfer, you should discuss, negotiate, and put in your legal contract your desire to use your surrogate's breastfeeding once the baby is born.

Touching Skin to Skin

From the moment of birth, babies react to touch. "Skin to skin" bonding is the ideal way to bond with your newborn; it involves holding them close to your bare chest. Early and frequent skin contact with you can help control your child's body temperature, stress threshold, and heart rate. It also activates oxytocin for the two of you. Give the baby a massage. Studies demonstrates that massage can increase parent-child connections while also alleviating newborns' tension and lessening parents' postpartum sadness. Get an online guide, read a book, or enroll in a class to find out how to massage your infant as effectively as possible. Maintain tight face contact and a lot of eye contact. Your infant can clearly communicate with you when they gaze up at your face and maintain eye contact. The infant will attempt to imitate your gestures and expressions right away. Spending a lot of time together face to face is the greatest method to maintain open communication.

Conversation with Your Kid

The sound of your voice does not calm or soothe your infant like it does. By talking to your child, you also extend an invitation to him to participate in your relationship. This aids him in organizing all of the new concepts he picks up from his surroundings. Your chats, reading aloud, and singing will be greatly enjoyed by the infant, especially when you mention or clarify things that you observe.

Participate in a Parenting Group

Specialty groups abound for parents of single children, adoptive and same-gender parents, parents of multiple children (where relevant), and many others. Joining a parenting group will give you a crucial support system and an opportunity to learn from other parents.

Chapter 5

Exploring Surrogacy and LGBTQ

Surrogacy is the only family-building option that allows LGBTQIA+ individuals and couples to have biological children. It's a process that requires medical and legal expertise, as well as strong emotional support throughout the journey. In recent years, **LGBTQ+ family-building options** have gained significant attention, marking a positive shift towards inclusivity in family dynamics. This emerging area focuses on the unique paths' LGBTQ+ individuals and couples can take to create their families. This chapter specifically addresses the needs and options available for LGBTQ+ individuals, shedding light on the various avenues they can explore. The options are growing, ranging from novel reproductive treatment.

As a result, many gay couples are now considering surrogacy and IVF as viable options to start their families. Similarly, adoption has opened doors for many to provide loving homes to children in need. Hence, this comprehensive exploration of LGBTQ+ family-building options reflects the evolving societal norms that celebrate diversity in family structures. Gay couples seeking parenthood have newfound hope through advanced fertility treatments. Donor insemination, where an egg is fertilized with a donor's sperm, stands out for its simplicity and success rates. Equally transformative is in vitro fertilization (IVF), a process of fertilizing an egg outside the body and implanting it in a surrogate or one of the partners.

Notably, IVF makes it possible for at least one couple to continue sharing genetics with the child. But these choices come with complicated ethical and legal ramifications. Navigating these aspects requires professional advice to safeguard the rights of everyone involved—the couple, the donor, and the surrogate. A complete grasp of various fertility procedures is essential for gay couples who are thinking about starting a family. It helps in planning ahead and provides a thorough overview of what's to come. Surrogacy is a significant pathway to parenthood for gay men, offering a chance to have a biological connection with their children. In this procedure, gestational carrier, also known as a surrogate, bears a child on behalf of the intended parents.

It can be done through traditional surrogacy, where the surrogate's egg is used, or gestational surrogacy, where the egg comes from a donor or one of the partner's female relatives. Around the world, there are vast differences in the legal framework around surrogacy; some nations are completely in favor of it, while others have strong restrictions. Gay couples need to understand these laws to navigate the process effectively. Also, surrogacy involves considerable emotional investment. Prospective parents and surrogates often develop deep, complex relationships. Financially, the process can be expensive, encompassing medical costs, legal fees, and compensation for the surrogate. So, gay couples must consider these factors and plan accordingly for a smooth and fulfilling surrogacy experience.

Embracing Your Special Family History

Your baby is finally here—the moment you have been waiting for a lifetime to experience! You may be wondering how your paths would cross again after this. Even though you have surely expressed your gratitude to your surrogate mother for the invaluable part she played in this trip. It might be challenging to predict with precision how your relationship will develop with your surrogate once the baby is delivered. It can be emotionally taxing to adjust to a new baby and the months that follow as a growing family and parent. For this reason, it's crucial to think through your post-birth plans for this already special relationship. Everything changes with birth, both for your surrogate and your family.

Finalizing the surrogacy process necessitates much planning and consistent correspondence. Naturally, communication dwindles once the baby is born since the parents are understandably preoccupied. But going through the postpartum phase without a newborn can be a challenging, abrupt change in responsibilities. Ultimately, all of your surrogate's other pregnancies ended with her taking care of a newborn. There won't be any feedings in the middle of the night, which some surrogates find to be a comfort, but for others, it can cause a confused range of feelings.

The intended parents' and surrogate's match meeting establish the groundwork for clear expectations and effective communication. It would be beneficial if you could talk about and share more about your preferences here.

Remember that during the process, these needs could alter and develop, which is why it's so important to speak with your match manager and surrogate directly. It's crucial to keep in mind that your surrogate can go through some degree of grief when the baby is delivered. She always knew this was your baby, so it's not the loss of a child; rather, it's the loss of the experience. Being a surrogate is a significant experience that alters her life as well. It's acceptable and healthy to have a range of emotions at the end of this process. During this phase, small gestures have a significant effect. It can mean the world to your surrogate if you just give her time to cuddle the baby. Snap a family portrait, or let her kids see the new arrival.

She might not request these items. Maybe she doesn't know how, or maybe she doesn't want to cause you any discomfort. By making the offer, you allow the journey to complete a circle and provide some closure for her and her family. Limits of ties between intended parents and surrogate mothers. Many potential parents may have genuine attachment-related worries at the beginning of the process. Is this, however, a justification for limiting communication? That, in my opinion, is what separates those who are not surrogates from those who are. It's evidence of the character and drive of many surrogate mothers as well as the efficacy of the screening procedure. Most intended parents and surrogates are able to find a comfortable communication level for all parties involved as the relationship develops and these worries fade, even after the baby is born.

Surrogacy Perception

In 1976, the first official surrogacy contract was drafted. The world and the United States have seen tremendous upheavals since then. It's time to address long-standing taboos that people may hold around surrogacy, given the tremendous amount we've learned about medical science and reproduction. Not everyone has accepted surrogacy to the same extent as it does now.

Although it was once viewed as experimental and frequently caused controversy, it has now been shown to be a valid substitute for family construction. Though thoughts on surrogacy remain controversial, the discussion is far more complex and varied, ranging from strong support to total misunderstanding. We'll discuss some of the widely held beliefs about surrogacy in this piece.

When you ask a surrogate why she decided to become one, her responses all have one thing in common: they want to experience parenthood with another family. The majority of surrogates decide to serve as a surrogate out of compassion and charity, even though they are aware of the possible risks and sacrifices involved. The goal of surrogacy is to enable another person to begin a family of their own. There are few deeds as unselfish as bearing a child for another family.

According to the most current survey, there are over 7.5 million infertile women in the United States alone who are between the ages of 15 and 44. Surrogacy is more than just a means of getting pregnant for many couples worldwide; for many, it's a second opportunity to become parents. Actress Elizabeth Banks talked candidly about her decision to use surrogacy back in 2012, when she supported family-planning alternatives and stood in solidarity with those impacted by infertility.

Surrogacy gives hope where many had given up on infertile women and their families. Fear of things they don't understand can exist. The surrogacy procedure is intricate, and you could feel confused or nervous if you don't know everything there is to know about the physical requirements. Many of the physical symptoms and difficulties associated with surrogacy are similar to those of a typical pregnancy. Fatigue, nausea, bloating, sensitivity, and other common symptoms might affect women.

There is always danger associated with medical procedures. To reduce your risk, make sure you meet the requirements and are in good enough condition to serve as a surrogate. Extensive research is the best approach to counteracting ignorance or bias, so make sure you do as much research as you can to become an informed expert on the subject. Whatever your opinions on surrogacy, it's undeniable that society has come a long way to allow a woman to bear a child for another family. The practice of surrogacy will continue to gain acceptance as society develops and learns.

Teaching Your Kids About Surrogacy

The level of involvement your surrogate has with your child in the future depends on what all parties feel comfortable with.

In other words, the relationship looks different for each and every match. Though it's wonderful when intended parents make the decision to keep their surrogate so involved, the relationship can be equally fulfilling without regular contact. While many surrogates recognize that it's not necessary, they nevertheless welcome and value the occasional photo and update. Furthermore, even though this will be covered throughout the surrogacy process, communication may deteriorate over time. Ultimately, the hope is that all parties will be able to look back on the surrogacy experience.

Even many adults find surrogacy to be a complex topic, so knowing whether and how to discuss it with your kids can be challenging. Being a surrogate involves family. Although you bear the brunt of the effort as the surrogate, your children and your entire family will be affected by the proceedings. For instance, your children may feel that you are less available to them due to your pregnancy and appointments, and they may feel a variety of feelings, such as joy and a desire to assist another family, jealousy, and longing for a sibling. It is nearly always advantageous to include your kids in the surrogacy process.

The extent of your children's involvement will probably start with a gentle introduction to the subject of surrogacy and progress to a more detailed explanation if a pregnancy is confirmed. This will depend on their age, maturity, and feelings regarding the surrogacy. Start by reading kids' books on surrogacy and various ways to start families. These novels explain the concept of surrogacy softly and aid in normalizing it. When you mention to your kids that you might wish to assist a different family in becoming parents in the future, find out what they think.

Inform your kids about the intended family and show them images as soon as you've discovered a match with the intended parents. After hearing their story, let them know you'll be attempting to assist them in becoming parents. To help you take photos to send to the intended parents, enlist the aid of your kids. Assure them that your family will always be remembered by mentioning that these photos will be featured in a unique storybook for the infant. Allow your kids to make drawings or letters for the baby's intended parents. Have your kids go to the intended parents' house if possible so they may see the place the baby will dwell.

Permit your kids to choose a unique toy for the infant and bring it to the nursery. To help your kids get to know the intended parents, take them out to supper as a family. Teach your kids how to discuss pregnancy and surrogacy with others. Provide them with answers that they may utilize when they get inquiries or remarks from friends, strangers, and classmates.

Your kids will gain a thorough grasp of surrogacy, its mechanisms, your motivations, and the baby's rightful place after following these stages. Engaging your kids in the surrogacy procedure will help them prepare for the birth of the baby and its eventual adoption by encouraging them to view surrogacy as a wonderful and unique gift.

Conclusion

Surrogacy is becoming more common in the US; between 1999 and 2013, gestational carrier cycles produced over 18,000 infants. In numerous other nations, surrogacy in any form is still prohibited. However, the number of people going abroad for surrogacy has dramatically increased in recent years. This is due to the prohibitively high cost of surrogacy—American organizations, for instance, frequently charge more than $100,000—as well as the challenges of locating surrogates in nations where payment is prohibited. A few of the nations that have grown in popularity for surrogacy are Thailand, Poland, Russia, Mexico, India, and Ukraine. Those who can afford it can also go to the United States. Surrogacy is a profound and legitimate way to become a parent, just like any other traditional way. The intensity of love, devotion, and the desire to raise and care for a child never change, even when the road may. Same-sex couples, couples battling infertility difficulties, and aspirant single parents can all fulfill their parental goals through surrogacy. Like any other expecting parent's journey, it entails meticulous planning, emotional investment, and a love attachment with the child.

The excitement and hard work that go into expecting a child, whether biologically or via surrogacy, are just as important and influential in influencing the lives of the parents and the new member of the family. There isn't always a straight road in the sometimes difficult and emotional process of surrogacy. There are many highs and lows throughout the process, from the moment you are paired with the surrogate until the baby is born. It's crucial to be ready for anything that might occur, but you also need to realize that you can't control every part of the trip and that you'll need to rely on your own judgment and leap of faith when making decisions. In summary, developing a strong bond with your newborn requires perseverance, creativity, and steadfast dedication. This process is enhanced by surrogacy, which brings a distinct layer to the mosaic of experiences that culminates in the unmatched parent-child bond. In part due to the media coverage of prominent celebrities using it, it has gained wider acceptance as a family-planning method. Having children for other people involves so much more than what the media portrays. You not only make the expecting parents' lives better forever, but you also become an inextricable part of something bigger than yourself.